Overcoming Fibromyalgia: Enjoying Life without the Pain and Fog of Fibromyalgia

KARA AIMER

Copyright © 2014 Plaid Enterprises

All rights reserved.

ISBN: 1508610673
ISBN-13: 978-1508610670

CONTENTS

1	Introduction	1
2	Theories On The Causes Of FMS	3
3	Symptoms Of Fibromyalgia	6
4	Proper Diagnosis	8
5	Treatment Of Symptoms	12
6	Sleeping With Fibromyalgia Pain	18
7	Dealing With Fibro Fog	22
8	Common Triggers Of Flare-Ups	25
9	Enjoying Life In Spite Of Fibromyalgia	27
10	Conclusion	29

INTRODUCTION

I want to congratulate and thank you for picking up this book, "Overcoming Fibromyalgia: Enjoying Life without the Pain and Fog of Fibromyalgia." Have you or someone you know been diagnosed with Fibromyalgia? If you are looking for a thorough compilation of information that can help you deal with all facets of fibromyalgia, from treatment options to support groups, you have found it. There are as many different ways to treat the symptoms of fibromyalgia as there are ways to treat any other condition. We will address many of the most successful treatment options as well as inform and discuss why they are successful. We will also discuss the problems you may face, and how to go about coping with this sometimes scary condition. The intent is to help you understand more about fibromyalgia; to begin, let's start with a few facts.

Fibromyalgia is a chronic pain disorder comprised of many other symptoms and associated issues in tow. The total complexity of this condition, also considered a syndrome, is such that it is often considered all consuming. The day to day lives of people dealing with Fibromyalgia can be affected on physical, mental and emotional levels. Fibromyalgia is a wide collection of symptoms and problems and is also known as fibromyositis, fibrositis and fibromyalgia syndrome or FMS. Due to several factors, FMS is not considered to fit the profile of 'disease'. So what does this mean exactly?

This means that diagnosing this syndrome can be very difficult at times. In many cases, people have been written off by both themselves and medical professionals as hypochondriacs. The symptoms can range from the individual as well as the strength with which each symptom manifests itself. The severity with which these symptoms present themselves can determine the way you are treated and the best ways to live with Fibromyalgia. The good news is there are more options than ever before, truly feasible options that can make a world of difference. This is obviously great news considering that children, teens, adults and senior citizens alike can have Fibromyalgia with the average being three percent to six percent of the population according to the National Fibromyalgia Association. Women do report being affected 10% more than men though, which happens to be the only preference presented. On average, women ages, 25 to 60 have a higher risk of developing Fibromyalgia than men of a similar age group. This also means that concerns like fibromyalgia during pregnancy are real. Although possible and manageable, it is important to discuss getting pregnant or being pregnant while you or a loved one suffer from FMS.

The symptoms can range from the commonly mentioned flu-like feelings of sore, painful achiness in the muscles to balance problems, migraines, and even morning sickness. The symptoms vary per person and can fluctuate depending on the time of day. It is very important to remember that there are ways to deal with whatever symptoms have presented. There are as many ways to treat as there are people who need the treatment. So what are the symptoms and what are the options? How can fibromyalgia even be diagnosed? So many questions, and luckily, so many answers. Thanks again for picking up this book, I hope you enjoy it.

Also, don't forget to grab your FREE Bonuses via the link at the end!

Now, let's get to it!

Disclaimer: This book is not intended to suggest or replace medical advice. The information contained in this work is intended as general information only. The information presented is not intended to diagnose, treat or cure any health issues or take the place of professional medical care. For persistent health issues or further questions, please consult your health care provider.

THEORIES ON THE CAUSES OF FMS

Natural Causes

The likely cause or explanation for why some people have FMS and why some have more symptoms than others is always under speculation and research. Various theories and research include the investigation into a natural chemical or hormonal imbalance. The belief in those cases is that the imbalances affect the way the nerves of the body signal. In other theories, the belief is that stress is the main trigger, causing the deep muscle pain, illness, trauma, fatigue and migraines that can all be associated symptoms of FMS. Stress is another seriously considered possible cause of FMS in that stress causes can cause insomnia, anxiety and other symptoms that could be considered to get the ball rolling for FMS to take root.

More prevalent is the idea that a set of many stressors could be the cause of several cases of FMS. In this research, the idea is that it may be a series of linked stressors or possibly multiple events that could be unrelated and even a combination of both physical and emotional, stressful events. The various options aside, the idea that multiple types of stress in any range of time could cause FMS. There is also research being done to find out if FMS is hereditary and if that means we can eliminate the gene or go into preventative treatment.

It is being considered that fibromyalgia may be similar to other rheumatic diseases that have a tendency to be passed genetically, mostly from a mother to daughter. The genetic traits that would be passed would be those that were related to the body's natural reaction to painful stimuli. If this should be the case, what is passed amplifies the feeling of most stimuli to an intensely painful level when most other people would not register any pain. There are some concerns that there is no actual way to pre-screen or predict who will get FMS because there is no explanation.

The Serotonin and Substance P link

Another indicator being seriously considered is lower quantities of serotonin because lower levels of this brain neurotransmitter are known to translate into a lower threshold for pain. Furthermore, women have been found to have much less serotonin than men, and women were found to have FMS in higher numbers than men.

There is also a Substance P and Serotonin link that is being heavily considered as a cause of FMS. The approach is multifaceted. The reduced effectiveness of the body's endorphins also means an increase in pain as endorphins are the body's natural painkillers. Working with the increase of the body's chemical known as 'Substance P' which amplifies pain signals make a sound argument for a cause of FMS.

Event and Physical Triggers and Causes

Further speculation includes the idea of micro trauma to certain muscles could lead to a chronic amount of fatigue and muscle pain. This consideration is sometimes tied to the idea that high amounts of stress coupled with poor physical condition can lead to FMS. Spinal cord injuries and/or brain trauma are also being considered as a link to FMS for certain people.

While all of these considered causes are being investigated and researched, they are still all pure speculation, and none has been proven as of yet.

There are many associated risk factors for Fibromyalgia:

- Again, females have a higher instance of having FMS than males.
- Menopause is another risk factor, attributed to the drastic loss of hormones like estrogen.
- Physical trauma, as stated above, is a risk factor, but all physical trauma is considered, in this case, such as brain or spinal cord injury and even in some cases surgery.
- Surgery is considered because of not only the trauma and stress on the body, but the emotional stress and other associated occurrences allow for surgery to be mentioned as a risk factor on its own.

Surgery would be considered an example of what is mentioned above, where multiple emotional and physical events lead to FMS.
- Lack of physical conditioning typically amounts to a weaker body and in some cases a weaker immune system, and thus the condition of your body could be considered a risk factor.

Overall, the causes and associated risk factors can seem like they are going around and around, but part of this is because scientists and researchers are continually working to identify the cause. The lack of a simple theory that sums everything up in a simple sentence shows the true complexity of FMS. While this may make it difficult to relay the information to friends, family and children, especially when you have to explain the condition to a child that is dealing with FMS directly or indirectly through you or a spouse, or another loved one or close relative.

Fibromyalgia is a serious condition though and should not be underestimated. Should you give in to the desire to give up and live with the fact that you are dealing with daily pain and other symptoms that seem to be unrelenting, you will not get better. There is a way to get better, many ways. That should not be forgotten in the large amount of annoyances and pain the condition can cause. In the vast majority of cases, one symptom can trigger another, and another and another until your body has gotten to the point where it can no longer work properly and repair damage to your tissues, which means you won't heal properly.

The body is extraordinary, even when it feels like your body is letting you down. Even with all the pain of FMS your body is still doing so much right that you want to keep going. Whether you are dealing with one symptom or many, there are answers and near-endless support out there for you. Symptoms can be treated well on an individual basis or en masse. There is no cure for FMS, but it is by no means considered fatal, and your quality of life can be improved upon and preserved with proper diagnosis and treatment. Let's take a look at the symptoms of FMS.

SYMPTOMS OF FIBROMYALGIA

Fibromyalgia is a condition comprised of the symptoms it produces. Due to this it can be very difficult to diagnose FMS accurately, and it can take a rather annoying amount of time. This is why it is so important to report ALL of your symptoms to your doctor, even if they seem irrelevant or unrelated. You are one of the biggest aids to diagnosing what you are dealing with. Doctors choose the tests they run based on the symptoms you exhibit and report.

The three most prevalently reported symptoms are so problematic that they do trigger other symptoms and affect the everyday quality of life people experience. These three symptoms include Pain, Exhaustion, and Fibro-Fog.

While the big three symptoms can be debilitating, they can also trigger other symptoms and it is of the utmost important to watch out for that and keep an open dialog with your doctor. Although family and friends try to relate, sometimes it can feel better to talk to others who are dealing with a similar situation as you. The use of a support group or online community dedicated to life with FMS can mean a lot of positive things, including access to treatments that you can talk to your doctor about that you may not have considered before. The overall breakdown of the most common symptoms is listed below. All are easily treatable but can lead to a misdiagnosis if you do not stick to your guns and work with your doctor in every relatable facet of your diagnosis and treatment. Muscular Issues, such as:

- Chronic muscle spasms, muscle pain, muscle tightness, possibly

even muscle stiffness from being stationary for an extended period of time or sleeping and severe muscle pain after exercising.
- Fatigue (moderate to severe)
- Fibro Fog – issues with concentrating, remembering things and even performing mental tasks and exercises that are typically considered simple things done by rote.
- Low energy
- Insomnia
- IBS (Irritable Bowel Syndrome: Bloating, alternating constipation and diarrhea, abdominal pain and nausea)
- Headaches, both tension headaches, and migraine headaches
- Tenderness in the jaw or face
- Anxiety
- Depression
- Sensitivity which can vary per person and can include Odors, bright light, noise, medications, cold and certain foods
- Numbness and Tingling in the extremities (arms, hands, legs, feet, face)
- Imagined Swelling of hands and feet
- An increase in the sudden urgency to urinate and/or frequency of urination
- TMJ dysfunction (Temporomandibular Joint Dysfunction) - a set of symptoms or issues associated with the joints of the lower jaw and the chewing muscles.

Many of these symptoms are associated with several different diseases and disorders. For example, Obstructive sleep apnea, Lupus, RA (Rheumatoid Arthritis), Hypothyroidism, Chronic Fatigue Syndrome, Lyme disease, Arthritis, and Malignancy are all conditions that share some of these symptoms in different arrangements. In certain other cases, Fibromyalgia is considered the secondary condition to something else. The symptoms are important indicators of the severity of your fibromyalgia, but it is also important to remember that things can change with time and the changing factors in your life. Certain things can aggravate your symptoms as well if you do not carefully take them into consideration. As with any other syndrome, changes that you experience should be reported to your doctor to keep your treatment not only current, but optimally effective. Your symptoms are the key to getting a proper diagnosis.

PROPER DIAGNOSIS

Diagnosing FMS can be a lengthy and troubling process, but is done through several means, although most prominently through the use of a particular physical exam. As no X-rays or other typical lab tests currently exist that will diagnose FMS with 100% accuracy and certainty, doctors rely on a series of tests that can indicate more accurately whether or not you have FMS. The process of diagnosing fibromyalgia can be extensive and in many cases have taken an average of 5 years to reach the point where the patient is successfully diagnosed with Fibromyalgia.

One of the worst things that a person who might have Fibromyalgia can do is to disregard their pain. Having your pain evaluated is an important step to finding out what is causing the pain. Ideally speaking the best thing you can do in regards to keeping track of and evaluating your pain on your own is to keep a journal of sorts. In your journal, make a note of every time you are experiencing pain. Include where you are experiencing the pain and a description of the pain as accurately as possible. Additionally, any other symptoms you experience should be written down with the date so that when you speak with your doctor, you do not have to rely on memory to describe your symptoms.

People with Fibromyalgia experience ongoing pain that is widespread. A lot of people find that the pain can vary from day to day, and perhaps the day that you do the pressure test you are not in a lot of excruciating pain. Let's be honest, a lot of us have called and made an appointment with the doctor, and once we finally get in there we feel fine. It is irritating because you know something is wrong, but it is almost like your symptoms are playing hide and seek with the doctor. Having this journal will verify your symptoms to the doctor. A fibromyalgia diagnosis usually means that the person diagnosed has been dealing with widespread, chronic pain in all four of the quadrants of the body for a space of time equal to three consecutive months or more.

While it is not necessary, the journal method is highly recommended, and templates can be found online. The website MyFoggyBrain is a great resource where you can find a journal template and plenty of information and a feeling of camaraderie. Furthermore, once diagnosed, your journal will still come in very handy.

In a lot of cases, the testing process has led to many different patients being misdiagnosed. Until recently, the best way to test for FMS has involved a physical examination that essentially tested 18 tender points on the body. A person who does not suffer from fibromyalgia will only feel pressure when these points are pressed. A person with fibromyalgia will experience pain. At the top of this list of tests are the tenderness point test and the FM/a blood tests. Depending on your doctor, you can have your tests done in a variety of ways. In most cases, a visit to a rheumatologist or another pain specialist is also made during the diagnosing stage.

The Old Way

With the tenderness points test, the patient has to test positive (feeling pain rather than just pressure) at 11 of the 18 tender or trigger points. These points are near joints though not the actual joints, and when pressed upon, a person who has fibromyalgia will feel pain rather than pressure. As with the origins or causes of fibromyalgia, why these points are painful to the touch (especially when the trigger points are about the size of a penny) is still not known. Even if you do exhibit pain at 11 or more of the 18 spots on the body, your doctor will still need to hear about your symptoms to confirm the diagnosis. It is important, however, to note that many doctors do not rely solely on the tender points test as the areas of pain can change for some.

If you show signs at a minimum 11 out of 18 trigger points, and the doctor takes a good look at your pain log or journal, you are likely to have to take a particular blood test. While the vast majority of lab tests are unhelpful when trying to diagnose FMS, there is one blood test, the FM/a blood test that can be a significant help. The FM/a blood test finds and identifies certain proteins or markers in the blood that are only produced by the immune system of those who have fibromyalgia. If your doctor does not mention it, and you are concerned, ask for the test. If it is right for you, he will do it, but he should discuss the option with you either way. A diagnosis leads to treatment and the start of you feeling better. So it can't hurt to ask right? At least no more than what you have written in your pain journal.

Afterward, your doctor may request a CBC, which is a complete blood count, as well as the FM/a. This test will see if you have any blood disorder, such as anemia by measuring the red cell and white cell count in your blood, the amount of platelets and your hemoglobin. Your kidneys and liver may also be tested so that the doctor can take a look at your blood chemistries. Your cholesterol, calcium, and sodium levels will also likely be tested. Thyroid tests may even be ordered to rule out hyperthyroidism and hypothyroidism, as well as other problems. To test the inflammation in your body, your doctor may also test your red blood cell sedimentation rate. In cases of fibromyalgia (and osteoarthritis) these levels are normal, but in cases where there are certain infections, Rheumatoid arthritis or other types of arthritis are present the test will be abnormal.

Should your doctor decide to test for the rheumatoid factor as well, or the ANA (anti-nuclear antibody) test you will know that they are eliminating other options such as Lupus and RA. While X-rays are not helpful in diagnosing FMS directly, indirectly they can show that you do not have certain types of arthritis or other inflammation issues. Fibromyalgia will not show results on an X-ray, so there is no need to worry if your doctor would rather not run that particular lab. They may be able to make the diagnosis without it and save you and your insurance the lab fees.

While this may sound like an intimidating amount of tests, it is important to remember that a diagnosis will mean treatment and a better quality of life. If you are worried that the tests will equal more pain, don't. After all even considering the list of tests your doctor may run to diagnose you, the great majority of the list is all done on a little vial of your blood. Cheers for technology, right?

The New Way

The May 2010 issue of Arthritis Care & Research published the findings of a study aimed at finding a newer and more effective way of diagnosing FMS in patients. The findings of this study created criteria for diagnosis that has already received the stamp of approval from the American College of Rheumatology and is considered to be a more effective and efficient method of diagnosis for FMS. The study was authored by Robert Katz MD, a professor of medicine at Rush University Medical Center in Chicago who is also a Rheumatologist. Dr. Katz says that this new method is not one hundred percent accurate all the time but is still considered to be a better testing option.

The new method involves the use of a pain index, in addition to the severity of key symptoms, to diagnose and quickly and properly treat patients with FMS. To test the pain, the patient is reporting, the doctor uses a 19-point pain index checklist. The patient is supposed to mark the body parts where thy have been having pain in the last full week. The symptoms checklist evaluates the levels of fatigue, cognitive issues, and unrefreshing sleep. The scale for these three symptoms is rated on a scale of 0 to 3 that measures the severity of each in an ascending order.

Considering the effectiveness, this new test is measured to have it is likely that the number of people diagnosed with FMS may at least double, possibly even triple. This is excellent news for those who have been misdiagnosed, or have been told they did not meet the criteria to be considered a person with Fibromyalgia. This increases the credibility of FMS, as more doctors who are not pain specialists will be able to properly diagnose and treat patients with FMS.

Thanks to the increase in ways to diagnose, it is easier to start treatment and improve the lifestyle of anyone with FMS. Treatments can vary based on preference, but there are so many treatments available that there is no reason to feel anything other than hope after receiving a positive diagnosis.

TREATMENT OF SYMPTOMS

There are several treatments available and a few of the top rated are listed below. There are more treatments available than I could list in this book, but that is a positive thing. There are a lot of different options out there, and no matter whether you are interested in Western Medicine as an option, energy work or homeopathic and organic food options, there are many ways to treat FMS.

Pharmaceutical Remedies

Currently, there are three medications that are FDA-approved and on the market to treat Fibromyalgia. In no particular order, these medications are Cymbalta (Duloxetine), Lyrica (Pregabalin) and Savella (Milnacipran).

Cymbalta is an antidepressant that works by increasing the activity of norepinephrine to stop pain signals from getting to the brain, and serotonin which also blocks pain. About 50% of those who give Cymbalta a try see an average reduction of pain by 35%. The depression and fatigue that are often associated with FMS are also relieved. Oddly though, the side effects that some people can experience with Cymbalta can include symptoms of FMS-like fatigue, insomnia, diarrhea, constipation, headaches, and nausea.

Lyrica is a seizure medication that is designed to stall and reduce the nerves sending pain signals to the brain. There are also benefits seen in regards to the quality of sleep those who take this medication experience. The associated side effects can include dry mouth, headaches, issues concentrating, sleepiness, dizziness, nausea, and vomiting. The addition of these side effects can be a significant problem for someone dealing with Fibromyalgia. The efficiency ranges from 30% to 40% in terms of pain reduction and only one-third of people actually see these results.

Savella is also an antidepressant and is the most recently approved by the FDA for the treatment of fibromyalgia. As with Cymbalta, the same statistics of 50% of users noticed a successful decrease in pain and depression of about 30% to 40%. The reduction of pain is not complete but still meaningful. The side effects can be symptoms you already have or may not have had beforehand, like diarrhea, headaches, stomach pain and insomnia.

Natural options

With fibromyalgia, you will most likely be taking a lot of medicines, it's just a fact of life. Many people who are just starting out on their quests rely on medicine along. However, some people who have had the disorder for a long time find fibromyalgia help through natural treatments — about 90% of those with fibromyalgia have tried some form of them by the end of their first year dealing with problems. Because there are few clinical studies on most of these treatments, the only way to see if any work for you is to try them. Here are just a few of the natural options people have found to alleviate the pain of fibromyalgia.

Aerobic exercise

Aerobic exercise is considered to be a great way to improve life overall for people with FMS. While it is definitely recommended that people start slow, the goal is to build up to 45 to 60 minutes each day of aerobic exercise that is low to moderately intense. Be warned, however, for many with FMS, it will definitely improve symptoms over time, but it will hurt initially. When it comes FMS and exercise, you have to stay motivated and get past the initial increase in pain to get to the lasting overall improvement to your daily life.

Cognitive behavioral therapy

CBT or Cognitive Behavioral therapy is a specific type of counseling aimed at changing people's reactions to various things. For people with FMS, this means changing the reaction to pain, outside stressors and triggers and how it affects them. Not only can this increase a person's coping skills, but it can improve the quality of sleep they have and help combat fibro-fog and fatigue. Some insurance companies do cover CBT, and for most people with Fibromyalgia, results are seen after an average of about 20 sessions. To get started, search for your local pain centers for information on CBT in your area or speak with your insurance provider. CBT works best when used with Biofeedback treatment.

Biofeedback

Biofeedback treatment involves the placement of sensors that will allow you to monitor and learn to control the processes of your body. After an average of 10 sessions, you could begin to control certain symptoms of your FMS, such as migraines and tension headaches, pain, and even morning stiffness. Though as with CBT, Biofeedback is not always covered by all insurance companies, there are many that do.

Physical therapy

Physical therapy is a great option for improving muscle pain range of motion and overall strength. Physical therapy can also help teach methods for pacing activities to keep from feeling worsened fatigue and pain during physical activity. The benefit of having a physical therapist who is familiar with your particular pain management issues and symptoms means personalized treatment and thus, better results. However, it is incredibly important to make sure that your physical therapist is trained and familiar with FMS. Without that knowledge, you could risk having much more pain throughout the beginning of your treatment.

Yoga

There are specific yoga classes that are geared towards people who have fibromyalgia. These classes frequently feature gentler poses like Child's Pose, and the well-known Downward Facing Dog pose. For about half of those with FMS, who take these types of yoga classes, approximately 30% reduction in pain, stiffness, and fatigue is to be expected. With minimal side effects, yoga is a great option. Staying motivated is key and finding a class taught by an instructor who knows about FMS is equally important. The only side effects are associated with doing poses that you are not ready for or doing them improperly. This can mean more pain until you have mastered the appropriate poses and mastered what you are doing.

Tai Chi

Tai Chi is a well-known form of martial arts that is individualized by the practices of deep, slow breathing and gentle, purposeful movements that flow seamlessly together. For those suffering from FMS, Tai Chi can mean an increase in endorphins, flexibility, muscle tone and strength, and a significant reduction in overall pain, anxiety, depression and better more restful sleep. In 2010, a study was conducted to measure the effectiveness of Tai Chi on fibromyalgia symptoms and an average of 80% of people with FMS experienced a marked improvement in their fibromyalgia related symptoms and pain. The study also found that 50% of people with FMS found any significant pain reduction when they only used stretching exercises. There are no known side effects of learning and practicing Tai Chi though the dedication and practice it requires may not be for everyone.

Acupuncture

Acupuncture uses the placement and manipulation of dry needles into the skin and the tissues just beneath. Studies on acupuncture have shown that correct use and application of acupuncture can alter a person's brain chemistry. The manipulation of the needles through twisting and other means a measurable level of endorphins to be released into the bloodstream. This increases a person's threshold for pain which means a decrease in pain. For those who are interested in the benefits of energy work to treat their FMS symptoms, acupuncture is considered to restore energy flow along specific energy channels which are called meridians.

Myofascial release therapy

Myofascial release therapy involves massaging the connective tissue to release the fascial restrictions. The tender points of the body are targeted, and the goal of the myofascial therapy is to work on reducing pain by working on the fascia found inside muscles, ligaments, bones and tendons. This treatment is performed by a physiotherapist who definitely knows what they are doing when helping a person with FMS. The physiotherapist massages your muscles to promote blood flow and lymphatic flow to restore function to the muscle as well as providing symmetry and making it easier and less painful to use the muscle.

Water therapy

Water therapy uses water exercises to decrease the pain and discomfort of exercise by using water as a buffer. An underwater treadmill can allow you to work out and increase your physical health and decreasing your physical pain. The warm water will soothe your muscles as you exercise and relieve much of the tenderness many people feel after working out. The water allows for buoyancy to come into play and also adds resistance to your workout, as well. Adding a therapeutic water class can not only give you more physical dexterity, but also strength.

Sensory Deprivation with a Flotation Tank

There are several ways to use sensory deprivation. A flotation tank is a favorite option for those looking to test the benefits of sensory deprivation. The floatation tanks allow for total quiet and darkness once the tank door is closed. The only thing you can feel and hear once in the tank is your own heartbeat and breathing. The tank has a solution of water and Epsom salt that is dense and allows for a person's body to float very easily. The solution is 93.5 degrees so it matches the temperature of your skin and will not trigger any sensitivity. This sensory tank experience is known as 'floating' and it offers a lot of benefits by putting the person in an almost meditative state. This allows for stress to be released, and a calming feeling that can reduce anxiety.

The use of herbs and supplements, especially Vitamin D are known to help as well, but it is important to discuss these with your doctor and nutritionist as some supplements and herbs can work against medications or even cause more severe reactions. There is also the use of chiropractic and osteopathic manipulation. It is all about customizing your treatment to suit you, your symptoms and your FMS.

Capsaicin Application for Fibromyalgia

Have you ever seen the scene in Orange is the New Black when Piper chews up the pepper to help with Red's aching back? She was doing that for the capsaicin. Capsaicin comes from pepper plants and is considered a natural pain reliever that is often put into plants. However, in developing countries, it is often chewed from the pepper and applied that way. More routinely, it's the active ingredient in a variety of over-the-counter sprays and lotions made available for pain relief. When applied to any painful area of the body, it stimulates the release of a chemical your body makes called substance P. As substance P is depleted, the pain seems to decrease for a time. Some cultures even make much of their foods spicy with real peppers as it acts as a natural pain reliever. There isn't much scientific proof to back that up, however. Capsaicin has been used for chronic pain in diabetes, cancer, and cluster headaches. It may also temporarily relieve fibromyalgia pain.

Melatonin Hormone

Melatonin is one of the miracle cures for those with insomnia and seasonal sleeping problems. It is a natural hormone found in the body and thought to be involved in promoting restful, uninterrupted sleep. Melatonin in pill or droplet form is often used as a sleep aid for those who may have jet lag or night terrors, but it has also been used for depression, chronic fatigue, and fibromyalgia. Again, the experts and scientists who have studied these claims say there is not enough evidence to support its use for the chronic pain of fibromyalgia. However, many people do get fibromyalgia help from natural and alternative treatments despite the lack of research support. Plus, sleeping more is a natural way for your body to heal itself and help you throughout the day. Consider this a good place to start if you can't sleep at night because of the aches and pains.

S-adenosylmethionine (SAMe)

Because SAMe is a naturally occurring substance throughout the body that your body produced and involved in many of the body's processes, its role as a pain reliever has been studied. There are even been some studies that have shown that those with fibromyalgia don't produce as much SAMe as those without the disorder do. SAMe has been studied for many different medical problems and has been shown to relieve depression and the chronic pain associated with osteoarthritis. Some studies show that taking SAMe may reduce fibromyalgia symptoms or even completely eliminate them – symptoms that interrupt daily life like pain, fatigue, and stiffness. The studies supporting the use of SAMe for fibromyalgia help are small, and not all have found a benefit, but it might be worthwhile to try it out for yourself if you have tried others within this list. More research is needed. SAMe is not found in food, but can be taken as a supplement in the form of a tablet that is typically available at most big box retailers and health food stores. You can also order it online.

SLEEPING WITH FIBROMYALGIA PAIN

Though we have talked about dealing with fibromyalgia pain, sleeping is truly a problem by itself that you need to tackle as a completely different villain. The sad truth is that over half of people with fibromyalgia experience significant sleep issues ranging from inability to fall asleep and stay asleep to daily fatigue to weird dreams from medications. You may have a hard time falling asleep or wake up multiple times throughout the night or you may fall asleep for hours at a time and miss your alarm clock. Maybe you don't spend enough time in the deeper sleep stages or maybe you dream so weirdly and can't get yourself out of them. Or you possibly suffer from all of it – making sleep something you crave and fear at the same time. It doesn't so much matter the precise sleep problem you have, but that you have one in the first place and it is severely impacting your daily life. Not getting a proper night's sleep will only aggravate your chronic pain and fatigue, and will also ruin the good days when you don't feel as much pain, but don't have the energy to do anything.

Finding a solution to your sleep problems will not cure your fibromyalgia, but it will reduce your pain and fatigue and give you a happier life. Plus, since those are arguably the most debilitating fibromyalgia symptoms and often the most annoying and damaging to your relationships, social life, and career, that may be consolation enough.

The Importance of Sleep When You Have Fibromyalgia

The value of sleep on a regular basis goes far beyond simply giving you a rest and allowing you some peace. It has significant psychological and biochemical importance that will impact not only your fibromyalgia, but your overall health as well. A few reasons your body needs a good night's sleep include:

- Sleep allows the body to repair damaged tissues which could lead to less overall pain for you.
- Dreaming promotes good physical and mental health, clearing up brain fog and helping with things like depression.
- Some essential hormones the growth hormone and sex hormones are secreted during sleep or shortly before waking, eliminating some of the other problems some people face – like unwanted hair growth.
- You concentrate better and are less fatigued with a good night's sleep. Lack of quality rest can induce what's sometimes called the fibro fog or the inability to focus and concentrate due to fibromyalgia's extreme fatigue.

Many researchers firmly believe fibromyalgia sufferers don't get enough deep sleep, which is the sleep that sustains us throughout the day – especially if we cannot get a nap. In the end, sleep researchers have identified three types of sleep for all people (the stages come in different timeframes depending on age): light sleep (stages 1 and 2), deep sleep (stages 3 and 4), and rapid eye movement or REM sleep.

If you don't spend enough time in the deep sleep stage, your body lessens that all important production of hormones that we talked about above. Decreased production of such hormones may increase pain in people with fibromyalgia as well as lead to many other problems.

Similarly, if you don't experience enough REM sleep, your body may produce less cortisol though the hormone, which controls blood pressure and blood sugar, may be released at any time during sleep. Remember that cortisol also can help with pain problems and sleeping issues. People with fibromyalgia may have low levels of cortisol, which contributes to their excessive fatigue.

Sleep is so critical to your health and your life. Here are just a few tips to help you out. Some of these are cross-references to other sections of the book so you might want to make notes and see what will cover a majority of your worst symptoms before picking one.

1. Anti-depressants. Some people find that low doses of tricyclic anti-depressants help achieve a deeper sleep. The drugs make people feel tired, and then fall asleep. However, it is just going to add to the amount of

medicine you take, so think about that before you make any firm decisions about what you do for your sleep. Talk to your doctor about possible side effects that may stop you from taking this – and make sure it won't mix with your current medications.

2. Don't watch TV, use your phone, or browse the Internet on your computer immediately before going to bed. These activities boost electrical activity in the brain, making it harder to fall asleep. It also tricks your brain into thinking that you are trying to fall asleep in the middle of the day because of the white light. Give yourself at least half an hour, if not more to wind down from the technology.

3. Get more exercise. Your pain and fatigue may keep you from exercising heavily or running any marathons, but light exercise may help you get a more restorative sleep. Make sure to give yourself time to heal and rest up before going to bed, or else you might stay up longer.

4. Herbal supplements. Valerian, kava kava, and melatonin are alternative medications that have helped some people fall asleep. Valerian helps with insomnia, kava kava also treats insomnia, in addition to stress and anxiety, and melatonin helps reset your body's natural rhythm, making it easier to fall asleep. These supplements can be difficult to find, so check at a health store or make your purchases online.

5. Mattress selection. This isn't just for people with fibromyalgia, but for all people who have a problem with sleeping. If you're not sleeping on a bed that encourages a good night's sleep, you might be in the market for a new mattress. There are a variety of mattresses available that may make a big difference in your quality of sleep including ones that change hardness and height so that you can deal with changing symptoms.

6. Prescription sleep remedies. There are a variety of FDA-approved drugs specifically for sleep disorders, including zolpidem (Ambien) and eszopiclone (Lunesta). Look out for the side effects of these, and try not to take them for long periods of time as they can be extremely addictive.

7. Simulate the breathing of sleep through meditation. This may "trick" your body into sleeping by taking slow deep breaths that mimic those of the deeper sleep stages. You'll feel relaxed and better able to fall asleep. There are a few different techniques to try through this – so you might want to go on YouTube and have a look around.

If you're experiencing sleep problems, talk to your doctor before you make any changes. It could be any number of things that you just need to change instead of trying something new. It might be your medication or the way you sleep. Whatever it is, together you will determine the best treatment options to give you the quality sleep you need to help curb your fibromyalgia symptoms.

DEALING WITH FIBRO FOG

Apart from the physical problems that one often faces with fibromyalgia, another huge problem that gets in the way of daily life is Fibro-fog. Fibro fog is the feeling of being in a haze – sort of like how it feels to be tipsy or high without the happiness that comes with it. This and related symptoms can vary from mild to extreme and may occur on and off depending on seasons, days of the week, sleep cycles, and even air quality. Overstimulation, stress, poor sleep, and certain medications can cause them to worsen.

Of course, not every fibromyalgia sufferer will experience all or even any fibro-fog symptoms, which include forgetfulness, memory difficulties, decreased alertness, inability to focus/stay focused, confusion, and/or lack of concentration.

How can you work to combat that fog? There's only so many lists you can make, alerts you can set, and post-it notes you can write. Here are a few more options to help you out:

Prescribed Medications

Certain medications that we have already touched on, such as Lyrica and Cymbalta, are used to treat the general symptoms and pain of fibromyalgia. However, they aren't targeted specifically to fibro-fog, but that doesn't mean they can't be used for it. Some people say that while it might not have fixed their fibro-fog, it fixed the situations that lead to having more fog. For example, many fibromyalgia sufferers are unable to get a restful sleep due to the physical pain they feel or their inability to sleep, in general. Their doctors may prescribe Ambien (zolpidem) or Lunesta (eszopiclone) to help with this symptom, this pill might help you feel good enough to sleep so that your mind has time to rest. The result of a rested mind? Less fibro-fog to deal with!

Mental Exercises

For some sufferers of brain fog from other diseases or treatments, brainteasers such as crossword puzzles, Sudoku, paint by numbers, and jigsaw puzzles can help to keep the brain active and decrease the symptoms of fibro-fog. This is because they require some thinking but aren't a situation where you need to really think. Games that require strategic thinking so that you can win (if that is important to you!) like Scrabble, bingo, chess, Parcheesi, checkers, and bridge help flex your brain and get the blood moving more, creating less fog.

Physical Exercise

Although it may seem contradictory, taking a break from your work and getting outside and moving will help your brain fog and your pain. Exercise will help to re-establish the natural neurochemical balance of the body and increase your natural "feel good" endorphins. This is helpful for fibro sufferers experiencing stress, anxiety, or depression. It will also just give you some time to clear your head – start counting the breaths you take or the steps as you walk or run and see if it makes a difference.

Acetyl-L-carnitine (LAC)

Acetyl-L-carnitine (LAC) is commonly used by psychologists and doctors to treat various mental disorders like bipolar disorder and depression. It also has shown some benefits for treating the mental dysfunction that occurs in our brains, causing us to get mixed up or confused. A 2007 study done on 200 patients indicated that acetyl-L-carnitine may help reduce pain and improve the mental health of some fibro patients.

Yoga and Mediation

According to a 2011 study, practicing yoga or meditation can increase cortisol levels which are a natural way to clear the head and stop the pain. Higher cortisol levels can reduce pain and increase "mindfulness," especially in female sufferers. It is best if you participate in at least two 75-minute yoga classes per week to gain the full benefits of yoga therapy.

Remember that the symptoms of fibromyalgia are as diverse as the patients and families who suffer from them. Unfortunately, there's not a one-size-fits-all treatment for fibro fog, especially because we all have something different on our minds. Try to slow down and lessen your load, especially at first or when you change medicines. This will definitely ease some of your problems. Remember to write things down, take advantage of recording options, and ask for clarification via email, if necessary.

Your best option is to work with your doctor or health care team to identify which therapies will help ease your symptoms and allow you to function better on a daily basis. It might actually take a little bit more time out of your schedule, but you will need to focus on your health before you can tackle anything else on your "to do" list.

COMMON TRIGGERS OF FLARE-UPS

The triggers for a fibromyalgia flare-up can vary from person to person and can be triggered by any variety of things from traveling to paying the bills. Here are a few of the most common triggers to get you started. Keeping your pain journal updated (though you may want to call it an FMS journal or log once you have been diagnosed) can help you identify the triggers of your flare-ups. This means that, in the future, you can avoid or pre-plan around an incoming trigger in the best manner for you and minimize the severity of the flare-up significantly.

Stress is one of the most obvious triggers for an FMS flare-up and is unlikely to be avoided. Stress can come from anywhere, anytime. If you know how to manage stress, you can deal with it before it engulfs you and causes a flare-up in your symptoms. There are things that you can do in a few minutes every day to alleviate the stress of day-to-day life before it can cause a flare-up like meditating, for example. Keeping on top of everything (as much as humanly possible that is) can also reduce the amount of stress in your life by drastic amounts.

Weather changes can cause a short term FMS flare-up and is one of the most commonly reported causes of flare-ups. Typically these flare-ups only last about a day or two, but they are associated with the barometric changes of a weather front moving through. Whatever method you use to treat and manage your pain, use it as you can and do not forget to record how you feel and what worked to relieve your symptoms in your pain journal. It is the best way to track changes and keep your doctor in sync with how you are feeling.

Over exertion is another trigger for flare-ups. This can happen even during the use of one of your chosen pain management options. If you push too hard or too fast, you can create a problem for yourself that can last a few days. Remember that gradually stepping up and carefully monitoring your progress will mean that you won't have to worry about overexertion, which can also damage your will to continue with your pain management and cause setbacks.

Illness and injury can not only trigger FMS but can trigger a flare-up of your FMS, as well. This is not to be taken lightly as even the common cold can cause a serious flare-up. Do not get discouraged, remember that there are options to ease the pain and speak with your doctor if you need to.

Traveling can cause a flare-up through various means. Depending on where you are going and how you are traveling there can be many concerns. Sitting stationary for a while can cause muscle stiffness for some. Depending on the starting and ending destinations, the elevations and weather may be drastically different and even the changes in temperature from one place to another can trigger a flare-up. Plan ahead as best you can and be prepared with whatever you know to be the most helpful method for you to manage your FMS.

ENJOYING LIFE IN SPITE OF FIBROMYALGIA

Fibromyalgia is a complex condition, and it requires a lot of active maintenance to stay on top of. Do not allow your FMS to take over your whole life. If you do, the anxiety and depression may start to take over. Take a class for your chosen treatment and get to know others around you who may have similar symptoms. One of the best ways to stay on top of your FMS is to get in contact with other people who can understand on a personal, intimate basis. In many cases, speaking to others can offer insight into new treatment options, excellent doctors, therapists and even just funny jokes to brighten your day. It is amazing what you can learn from someone on the same page.

Use of forums and online support groups can be a very big aid as well, such as:

- http://www.dailystrength.org/c/Fibromyalgia/forum
- http://exchanges.webmd.com/fibromyalgia-exchange

These are active communities of people trading the information that has helped them and how as well as general messages and information that they found relevant. There is a massive online presence for FMS and the benefit of this is that you have tons of support that you can carry around in your pocket or bag and access with your phone, tablet, laptop, etc.

There are plenty of blogs on this topic, as well. For example, the best Fibromyalgia related blogs are available on the following lists of the best fibromyalgia blogs. The first list will take you to a list of the top 16 FMS blogs. The second will take you to the list of the top 100 FMS related blogs.

These meet the author's criteria for being entertaining, helpful and resourceful. Follow some of them and see what they are about:

- http://www.healthline.com/health-slideshow/best-fibromyalgia-blogs
- http://www.b12patch.com/blog/fibromyalgia/100-best-sites-for-fibromyalgia-or-chronic-fatigue-information/

CONCLUSION

It is important once again to remember that although fibromyalgia is a lot to handle, it can be handled. I hope that you have found this book to be resourceful, informative and encouraging. Help get yourself diagnosed. Find the treatments that work for you. Customize your treatments to suit your needs and how you want to live your life with FMS. Join a community and help yourself and others by sharing your story. If you are looking into FMS for a loved one, understand the complexity of this condition and use the information that you have learned to be a positive source and an aid for their treatment.

Thank you for picking up this book! I sincerely hope the information contained will help you to understand more about Fibromyalgia and FMS, as well as how to approach the treatment of symptoms.

The next step is to put into practice the methods and employ the strategies we've discussed here to begin taking your life with FMS to the next level in spite of this unfortunate condition! Only you have control over where your dreams will take you.

Finally, if you enjoyed this book, please take the time to share your thoughts and post a positive review on Amazon. I would greatly appreciate your support!

Thank you and good luck!

Kara Aimer

Don't forget your FREE Bonuses at: www.plaid-enterprises.com/fibro

COPYRIGHT NOTICE

© Copyright 2014 by Plaid Enterprises - All rights reserved.

This document is geared towards providing exact and reliable information in regards to the topic and issue covered. The publication is sold with the idea that the publisher is not required to render accounting, officially permitted, or otherwise, qualified services. If advice is necessary, legal or professional, a practiced individual in the profession should be ordered.

- From a Declaration of Principles which was accepted and approved equally by a Committee of the American Bar Association and a Committee of Publishers and Associations.

In no way is it legal to reproduce, duplicate, or transmit any part of this document in either electronic means or in printed format. Recording of this publication is strictly prohibited and any storage of this document is not allowed unless with written permission from the publisher. All rights reserved.

The information provided herein is stated to be truthful and consistent, in that any liability, in terms of inattention or otherwise, by any usage or abuse of any policies, processes, or directions contained within is the solitary and utter responsibility of the recipient reader. Under no circumstances will any legal responsibility or blame be held against the publisher for any reparation, damages, or monetary loss due to the information herein, either directly or indirectly.

Respective authors own all copyrights not held by the publisher.

The information herein is offered for informational purposes solely, and is universal as so. The presentation of the information is without contract or any type of guarantee assurance.

The trademarks that are used are without any consent, and the publication of the trademark is without permission or backing by the trademark owner. All trademarks and brands within this book are for clarifying purposes only and are the owned by the owners themselves, not affiliated with this document.

CPSIA information can be obtained
at www.ICGtesting.com
Printed in the USA
LVHW012101070721
692086LV00010B/1092